Peter Fincham has appeared radio programmes, talking a analysing and describing i matters, he is not married ~~but~~ lives with his girlfriend, Empress, and their three piglets. In 1982 his contribution to society was officially recognised when the Queen decorated him with four coats of emulsion and some cork tiles. He died in November 1984 and went on to work for the Post Office.

Patricia McGrath's interest in psychosexiosociochemical therapy stems from being asked what it means on *Call My Bluff*, one of literally hundreds of TV and radio programmes on which she has appeared, talking about sex, advising, counselling, analysing and describing it. She's the editor of several magazines, including *Sex Weekly*, *Sex Fortnightly* and its equivalent for married couples, *Sex-Just-About-Once-A-Monthly*. She wrote her doctoral thesis on earthworms . . . though a lot of them got killed going through the typewriter.

Ian Moore is the pseudonym of Swedish sexologist Axel Knobhardt. He has written many books on sexual matters, most notably *Vaginal Orgasm: Myth or Musical Instrument?* and *Where there's Muck there's Brass*—an investigation into the use of trombones in pornography. Ian Moore is an expert in many fields, and quite good in a bed too. He has been married and divorced 27 times and now lives in the top drawer of a filing cabinet.

'Bilivest thou in sexe before mariage?'
'Not if it delayes the ceremonye . . .'
Geoffrey Chaucer

Illustrated by Nigel Paige

Sex

MADE SILLY

Patricia McGrath, Peter Fincham and Ian Moore

CENTURY · LONDON

Also available
Food Made Silly
Money Made Silly
Skiing Made Silly

Design/Gwyn Lewis
Graphics/Ian Sandom

First published in Great Britain in 1985
by Century Hutchinson Ltd, Brookmount House,
62–65 Chandos Place, Covent Garden, London WC2N 4NW

ISBN 0 7126 1017 0

Filmset by Deltatype, Ellesmere Port
Printed in Great Britain in 1985 by
Hazell, Watson & Viney Ltd., Aylesbury, Bucks

Authors' Note

Sex Made Silly is a book for all the family, so we'll be doing our best to avoid four-letter words such as 'vagina', 'penis' and so on (though this is in fact two separate two-letter words); also such Anglo-Saxon terms as 'rectum' (from the Latin—'rectus') and 'pornography' (from the Greek).

When we want to refer to a 'c---' we'll call it a 'c--t' or possibly a '-un-'. Whatever else, we'll be careful not to put 'c--t' and '-un-' together to form '----'. The same applies to '----' (otherwise known as the 'f' word) and '----' (which we'll be referring to by its popular name 'J. Arthur Rank').

It may be that you regard this attitude as prudish and narrow-minded. In a way I don't blame you. It's just that we've been warned by our editors that the minute one of these naughty words slips in they'll stop printing. Though why the fuck they

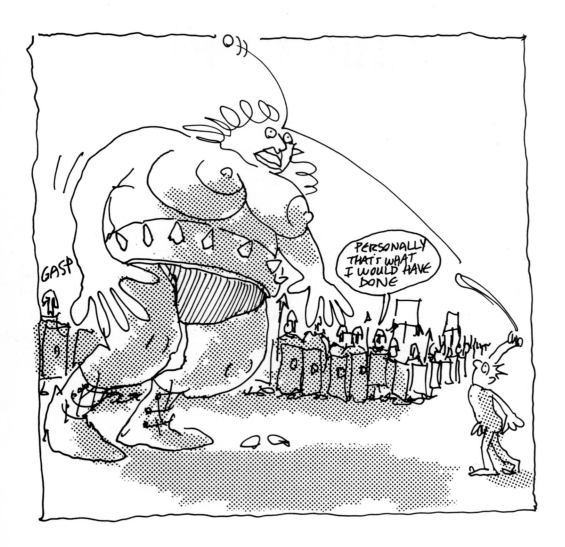

The Bible

Unauthorised Version

Genesis

In the beginning was the Word . . . and the Word was Made Flesh. I'm sorry . . . that's two Words. The Word was God. And God was the Word. The Word that was God, was God. And the God that was the Word, was the Word. So it all turned out rather well in the end.

2/ All was empty, shapeless, formless and lifeless, and God looked about him saying 'Hey, this could be Coventry on a wet Sunday!'

3/ All was dark. Everywhere complete blackness loomed. God moved silently through the darkness . . . and eventually stubbed his toe on the Universe.

4/ 'Let there be light,' said God. And there was light.

5/ 'Let there be sky and earth,' said God. And there was sky and earth.

6/ 'Let there be Eden,' said God. And there was Eden.

7/ 'Hey, this is a good trick,' said God. 'Let there be an attractive masseuse, a chilled bottle of bubbly and a deep-pan pizza!' And there were all these things . . . only the pizza was a bit slow arriving due to staff shortages in the kitchens.

8/ And then God created the animals and birds in the forest, and the flowers in the fields. He created the fish. Then he created the sea, because a lot of the fish were dying.

9/ And then he created Adam in his own likeness. And he saw that Adam was lonely, so he said to Adam, 'I will make you a partner'. So they set up God Associates.

10/ And while Adam was asleep, God took a rib from his chest, and Adam said 'Aaaaaaaaaaaaaaaaarrrggghhhh!!! What the f★★★!!??' And God made Eve in his own likeness . . . but that was no good . . . he wouldn't know her from Adam.

11/ And God said to Adam, 'Go forth and multiply.' So Adam went forth and multiplied and was away for six hours. 'Stupid git,' said Eve.

12/ And when Adam returned God tried again, only this time less subtly—'Shag her, then!'

13/ And so Adam and Eve discovered sex, and all that went with it: guilt, misery, jealousy, VD, divorce, duels at dawn, St Valentine's Day, Penthouse Pets, babies, war, Rupert Murdoch, expensive restaurants, agony aunts, the London Rubber Company, the Liberal Party, changing the sheets, more guilt, dirty weekends, taking the phone off the hook, Brewer's Droop, leather jockstraps, watching schools' hockey on the telly, Vaseline, continental holidays, special clinics . . . and some more guilt just in case.

Authors' Second Note

Sex Made Silly will, hopefully, be of equal value to both male and female readers, and the authors have taken great pains to ensure a balanced point of view. At the same time we don't want to keep talking about his (or her) sexual identity, or the way she/he feels about him/her/it or whatever.

So after thinking about the problem for a couple of minutes, we've decided to stick to the male gender, except when we use the female one. In either case they're completely interchangeable. If we write a sentence like 'At this stage he inserts his penis into her vagina' (which we won't anyway—see *Authors' First Note*) it might just as well mean 'She inserts her penis into his vagina.' By the same token 'If your teenage daughter gets pregnant' is the same as 'If your teenage son gets pregnant' (though rather less alarming).

The last thing we would want people to think is that *Sex Made Silly* is sexist or chauvinist in any way. Certainly our wives didn't think this when they were typing out the manuscript—bless them!—and I don't see any reason why our readers should think so either.

Just How Good In Bed Are You?

A survey of sexual performance, knowledge and understanding conducted by Baron Roger du Rex, French man of letters.

(1) Do you make love to your partner . . . ?
    (a) once a night.
    (b) once a fortnight.
    (c) once every five minutes.
    (d) once.

(2) How do you react to this statement: 'Buggery is a criminal offence punishable with life imprisonment?'
    (a) The law's an ass.
    (b) I don't believe you.
    (c) Sorry, officer—I was just bending down to tie up my shoelaces.

(3) Do you think oral sex is . . . ?
    (a) talking about it.
    (b) talking about it with your mouth full.
    (c) having your cake and eating it.

(4) How old were you when you had your first sexual experience?
    (a) 12
    (b) 16
    (c) 18
    (d) 69
    (e) age now plus 3 hours.

(5) Which of the following have you ever said to your sexual partner?
- (a) You're the only man I've ever loved.
- (b) You're the only woman I've ever loved.
- (c) You're the only sheep I've ever loved.
- (d) Not tonight, I've got a headache.
- (e) Not again, I've got an earache.
- (f) How was that?
- (g) How was what?
- (h) Not out.
- (i) Not in.
- (j) Not that shape.

(6) Do you make love . . . ?
- (a) with the light on.
- (b) with a hat on.
- (c) with a hard on.

(7) Would you describe yourself as . . . ?
- (a) an Alpha.
- (b) a Beta.
- (c) or wouldn't you want to be compared to any particular continental car?

(8) Do you smoke after intercourse?
- (a) yes.
- (b) no.
- (c) I don't know, I've never looked.

(9) Are you . . . ?
     (a) a leg man.
     (b) a breast man.
     (c) a milkman.
     (d) a woman.
     (e) a man's man.
     (f) a gentleman's gentleman.
     (g) a ladies' man.
     (h) a ladies' lady.

(10) How interested in sex are you?
     (a) very.
     (b) slightly.
     (c) hardly.
     (d) not at all, now please go away and stop bothering me you dirty little Frenchman.

(11) Do you prefer it . . . ?
     (a) from the back.
     (b) from the front.
     (c) from the side.
     (d) or are you perfectly happy with your new haircut?

(12) How far did you go on your first date?
     (a) necking.
     (b) groping.
     (c) all the way.
     (d) Newport Pagnell.

Sex and Evolution

According to a man who was not made Poet Laureate in 1984, sexual intercourse was invented in 1963. This isn't actually true (see *Sex and History*) as sexual intercourse has been around for many millions of years—in fact a good deal of animal and plant life was reproducing itself long before Man was even a twinkle in his Ape-father's eye.

Not all of this reproduction involved sex and indeed there are still life-forms which have rejected a male-female divide (e.g. amoebae, slime funguses, women's collectives etc.).

Simple one-cell animals reproduce themselves by dividing into two, an elegant and rather obvious way of expanding the

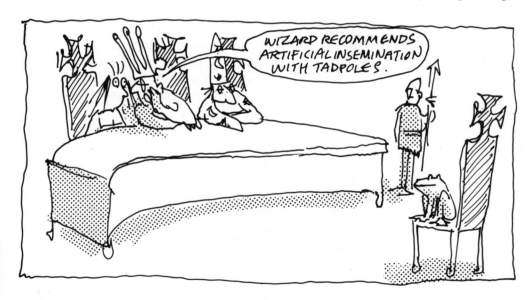

population which at least cuts out the need to find a partner and go to discos on a Friday night. In fact it is not clear why the higher animals and plants have elected to go in for the complicated business of sexual reproduction though arguably, however bad your sex life is, it's better than sitting at home and chopping yourself in half whenever you feel a bit broody.

Sex and Animals

Ever since Charles Darwin conclusively proved that man was descended from the apes . . . when he jumped into a tree and peeled a banana with his feet . . . there has been a close examination of the similarity in sexual habits between man and animals.

There are also important differences. Human adults generally mate lying down and face-to-face, whereas mosquitoes mate in flight. Humans very rarely mate in flight. There are exceptions, of course . . . pilots and stewardesses, for instance . . . but this is dangerous and quite often cramped.

Similarly, toads take twenty-four hours to complete sexual intercourse, whereas humans can take anything from twenty-four seconds to twenty-four years. And the female stickleback can be fertilised by any number of male sticklebacks . . . whereas the female human is very rarely fertilised by sticklebacks at all. Unless it's a really butch stickleback who's just showing off to his friends. Human mating usually requires one male and one female, though there are occasions when a second man is present . . . nervously hiding in the wardrobe.

Sex and Food

Finally, a lot has been written about the link between sex and food, though the only member of the animal kingdom to have successfully combined the two is the female black widow spider, which has been known to eat the male just after copulation. Perhaps as modern day feminism gains support throughout society this idea will catch on in the human world. This would certainly be an ideal solution for the problem of post-coital embarrassment, since if the man is eaten immediately after sex it saves him having to think of excuses as to why he has to leave straightaway or what he's going to say to his wife when he gets home.

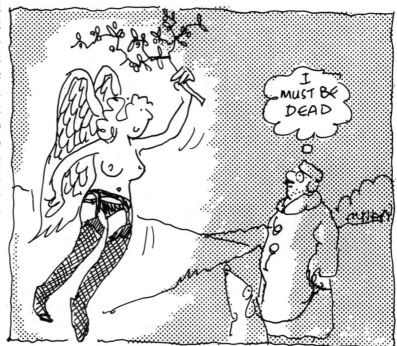

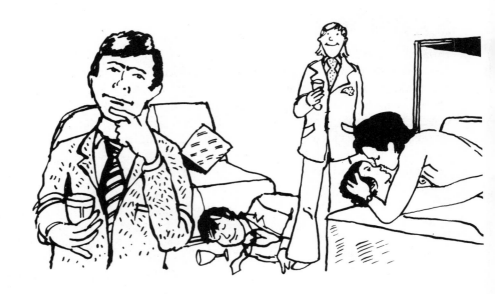

Body Language

Ten years ago nobody had heard of this curious concept, but now it's all the rage, and everywhere you go people are talking about body language, discussing it, analysing it—and all without saying a word.

According to the experts who invented the idea, the posture a person adopts provides all sorts of hidden clues to his personality, intentions, size of beer gut etc.

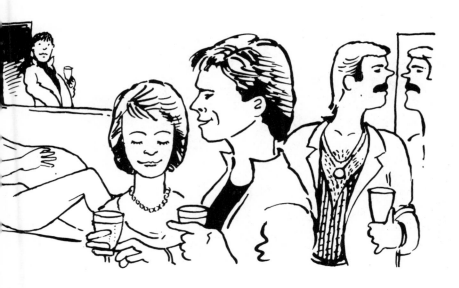

● Does he stroke his chin with his hand while you're making an interesting point? He's probably the thoughtful, responsive type.

● Does he flick his hair back off his forehead and catch his reflection in the mirror at every opportunity? Watch out—he may be suffering from an excess of vanity.

● Does he slouch in a doorway and dribble out of the corner of his mouth? He's drunk.

Look carefully at the illustration and see if you can spot all the hidden body language, sexual or otherwise, that's going on at this typical cocktail party.

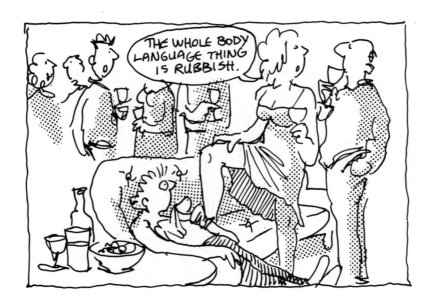

● She looks down while he's speaking to her:
(a) She's shy but secretly flattered
(b) She's aware of his signals and confident of the situation but wants to make him work hard
(c) He's just been sick on the floor.

● His hand resting on her forearm: could he be trying to tell her something?
   His other hand up her skirt: yes!

● He's twiddling his earlobe while she's talking. This is a nervous gesture thought to indicate a reluctance to listen to someone . . . or to hear something unpleasant like her saying 'Stop twiddling your earlobe, you pillock!'

Other typical 'body language' gestures include:

Legs crossed (male) A 'closed' gesture which puts a woman off. It means 'Don't come near me' or 'I've got a hard-on.'
Keeping your legs crossed is commonest among people sitting opposite each other on trains.

Fingers crossed This is commonest among people who haven't bought tickets on trains.

Leaning back, legs apart (male) A laid-back posture which can tell a woman quite a bit about you:
(1) You're relaxed
(2) You're pissed
(3) You're dead
(4) All of above.

Leaning back, legs apart (female) Indicates relaxation and confidence. This can be a 'come-on' to a man, particularly accompanied by a pointing-to-the-vagina gesture and the words 'Fuck me, fuck me!'

Hands clasped together behind the head A common gesture indicating that you are sitting opposite a terrorist with a rifle.

Flared trousers Either he thinks fashion stopped in 1975 when they went out or he's determined to say 'I told you so' when they finally come back in.

Medallions Worn by men with hairy chests and cheap aftershave as a sign of impotence.

Toupée Some girls go for the tall, dark stranger with a full head of hair and an air of mystery—the mystery being that last time you saw him he was completely bald.

Sex: Where To Have It

Ask most men what is the best place to have sex and they will surely reply, 'In between a girl's legs.' But nowadays even that puerile answer seems outmoded. In 1902 a survey of 10,000 married couples showed that they would only have sex in the marital bed . . . Of course the queue was endless . . . so people started being more adventurous about where they would do it.

Open Air Making love in the great outdoors is natural, healthy and exhilarating . . . and is not to be confused with making love on the grate indoors which leaves a series of lines on your bottom. Having it off in fields is a very good idea, especially in a newly sown field where the humping motion will frighten the birds. This makes it very popular with farmers, though it can be disconcerting when halfway through the act your bird walks away.

Planes Cramped and awkward: if God had intended us to have it off while flying he'd have made us dragonflies.

Cars Sexual acts are best suited to British cars as these are stationary longer than most as you wait for the AA to arrive.

Public telephone boxes Congratulations if you can manage to have it off in a public telephone box . . . but let's face it, it's slightly easier than making a phone call.

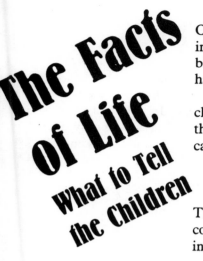

The Facts of Life

What to Tell the Children

Children have the great advantage over adults of being highly intelligent. It is vital therefore when explaining about the birds and the bees to explain also why a bee would want to have it off with a bird in the first place.

It is also important to choose the right moment to tell your children about sex. It should be after they're born but before they're married. Timing is paramount, otherwise it could cause some embarrassment. For example:

> 'Son, I want to tell you about the facts of life.'
> 'Not now, daddy, I'm on the job!'

This indicates that you are too late, too unobservant and completely stupid. But don't worry, you probably only exist in works of fiction.

This is probably the best way to explain the mystical process of reproduction to kids in a direct, scientific, honest way . . .

● Inside Mummy there is a little blob of stuff.

● This is called a 'blob of stuff'.

● Inside Daddy there is also a blob of stuff. This is completely different from the blob of stuff in Mummy . . . because it's got a tail on it.

● This is called 'another blob of stuff, with a tail on it'.

● It has a tail on it so it can
  (a) draw attention to itself.
  (b) wag it up and down when it's happy.
  (c) point to where the pheasant you've just shot has landed.

● a blob of stuff

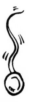

● another blob of stuff with a tail on it

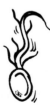

● When these two blobs of stuff come together they start growing like this

● Then they grow a little more like this

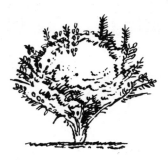

● And finally they grow into a gooseberry bush.

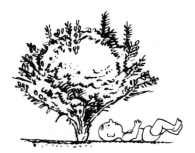

● And then one night a stork flies along and puts a baby underneath it.

● There's also a few other bits and pieces, but you needn't worry about them as they're all revoltingly smelly and rude and disgusting.

The Sex Made Silly

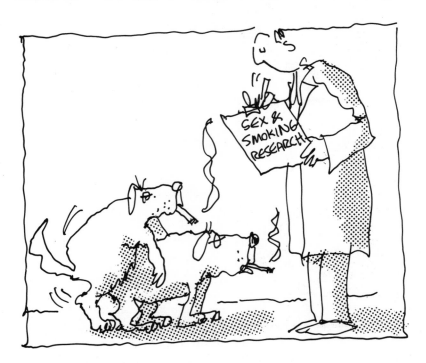

Sex Survey

> '*Male sexual response is far brisker and more automatic, and can be easily triggered by things—like putting a quarter in a vending machine.*'
>
> *Alex Comfort*

If you suffer the same problem as Mr Comfort, i.e. being turned on by the sight of vending machines in action, you may be interested in the results our research team have come up with:

● A recent survey revealed that between the ages of 15 and 25, *98%* of the average male's waking hours (and all of his sleeping hours) are spent thinking about sex. What was thought about during the other 2% was not revealed, but some of it must have been spent dreaming up silly answers to questions asked in surveys.

● A special *Sex Made Silly* poll concluded that in fact *100%* of the average human being's time was spent thinking about sex. But then it was realised that the poll was based exclusively on the responses of the authors of this book, at the time they were writing it . . . so possibly it wasn't statistically relevant.

● We decided to ask people how often they had sexual intercourse. Answers expressed as a percentage (because we only asked 7 people):

2% said once a fortnight, but that once was now, so could we ring back later.

10% said twice a day or as often as they could get it, whichever was the lesser.

15% said never, but call back when the Mother Superior isn't listening.

2% said not you again, we haven't finished yet.

11% said they would call the police if we didn't go away.

20% said three times a day, after meals, with a brush recommended by their dentist, pardon.

15% said six times a week . . . no, this *is* the Mother Superior.

2% said they couldn't speak now, they had their mouth full.

13% said they didn't know.

10% said they didn't care, but thought it important that percentages added up to 100.

17% said they didn't care, and didn't care whether the percentages added up either.

2% phoned up to say they had just finished, and you can see now why we only do it once a fortnight.

100% of the research team said this is dull, let's go back home and make up the results.

50% of the research team suggested that they have sex with the *other* 50% instead, and make up the results in the morning.

50% of the research team said you must be bloody joking . . .

YOUTHFUL, 45-ISH, NON-SMOKING PROFESSIONAL MALE NECROPHILE SEEKS FEMALE MEMBER OF EXIT FOR LONG-TERM RELATIONSHIP. BOX 367

INDECISIVE MALE LACKING IN CONFIDENCE SEEKS TALL BLONDE GIRL FOR SERIOUS RELATIONSHIP . . . OR SMALL DARK GIRL FOR CASUAL RELATIONSHIP. BOX 064

NERVOUS, SHY, AGORAPHOBIC SEEKS SIMILAR FOR CLOSE RELATIONSHIP. BOX 402

INCREDIBLY CONCEITED SMUG BASTARD WHO DOESN'T REALLY NEED TO ADVERTISE (OWN HOUSE, OWN CAR, GRADUATE, PROFESSIONAL, LONDON, RICH, GOOD IN BED, WELL-INFORMED, LIKES THEATRE, FILM, OPERA, SPORTS, MUSIC ETC.) SEEKS WOMAN TO BORE THE PANTS OFF. BOX 129

INTELLIGENT, ATTRACTIVE MALE SEEKS PIECE OF BENT METAL TO START VINTAGE CARS. NO CRANKS, PLEASE. BOX 345

BROTHER OF FUTURE KING SEEKS TARTY BIT FOR CASUAL SEX. GENUINE OFFERS ONLY. CONTRACT WITH NATIONAL NEWSPAPER USUAL BUT NOT ESSENTIAL. BOX 721

6'4" FLUENT RUSSIAN-SPEAKING PROFESSOR OF GENETICS, INTERNATIONAL BRIDGE PLAYER, BEST-SELLING AUTHOR, KARATE EXPERT, COMMANDO-TRAINED, CHESS GRANDMASTER AND QUALIFIED OBSTETRICIAN SEEKS SIMILAR. BOX 491

NOT VELY STLONG CHINESE LICKSHAW-PULLER LOOKING FOR MRS LIGHT. BOX 105

ATTRACTIVE, SINCERE MALE WITH OEDIPUS COMPLEX SEEKS 'FATHER FIGURE' FOR MEANINGFUL BUT SHORT RELATIONSHIP. BOX 429

Sex and History

10,000 BC ●	Dawn of civilisation.
●	'Early man' characterised by low forehead, jutting chin and Brut aftershave.
6000 BC ●	Cave drawings found in parts of Europe and Asia . . . mostly drawings of antelopes and buffalos . . . little evidence of sex, apart from occasional naked women in Cave Three.
5000 BC ●	Early woman announces to early man that she is late.
4999 BC ●	Birth of early baby.
3000 BC ●	Centuries pass . . . entire civilisations come and go—first the Sumerians, then the Phoenicians, then the ancient Egyptians, then the Sumerians again—they've forgotten their scarf.
1000 BC ●	Beginnings of Greek civilisation, undoubtedly the greatest the world has yet known.
427 BC ●	Birth of Plato, famous philosopher and inventor of the platonic relationship, which proves a great success.
426 BC ●	End of Greek civilisation.
250 BC ●	Invention of Roman bath . . . huge advancement in personal hygiene and consequently more sex . . . sales of Brut aftershave decline.
●	Invention of Roman Forum, innovative magazine in which people write in with questions about foot fetishism, premature ejaculation etc.

28

55 BC ● Romans invade Britain; after initial fighting the Romans and British agree to live peacefully together.

122 AD ● Construction of Hadrian's Wall to keep out ghastly hordes of Picts, Scots and Celtic supporters.

406 AD ● Romans announce that they are leaving and that the British will have to fend for themselves . . . they decide to still be friends, though, and meet once a month or so for lunch to catch up on each other's news.

500 AD ● Beginning of the Dark Ages, marked by a series of invasions . . . first the Anglo-Saxons . . . who sailed over in their boats, picked a random village on the English coast, grabbed whatever they could lay their hands on then sailed home again, thus inventing the Duty Free day trip.

● Simultaneous invasion by masses of visiting Jutes, which goes on for ten years, excluding time added on for stoppages.

● Pound sinks to new low and England becomes a tourist's paradise; Vikings, Danes and other Scandinavians pour in, bringing tales of free love and expensive lager.

1066 AD ● Norman Conquest, in which a chap called Norman irritates everyone by seducing all the prettiest girls.

1100 AD ● Beginning of Middle Ages, in which everyone loses interest in sex anyway.

THE KINGS OF ENGLAND

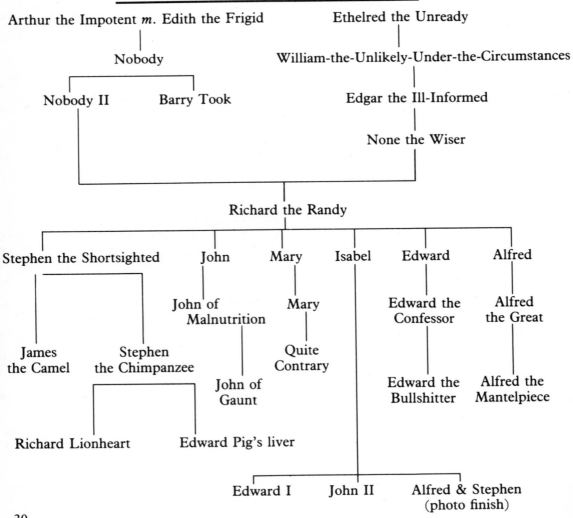

Arthur the Impotent *m.* Edith the Frigid

Ethelred the Unready

Nobody

William-the-Unlikely-Under-the-Circumstances

Nobody II   Barry Took

Edgar the Ill-Informed

None the Wiser

Richard the Randy

Stephen the Shortsighted   John   Mary   Isabel   Edward   Alfred

John of Malnutrition

Mary

Edward the Confessor

Alfred the Great

James the Camel   Stephen the Chimpanzee

Quite Contrary

John of Gaunt

Edward the Bullshitter

Alfred the Mantelpiece

Richard Lionheart   Edward Pig's liver

Edward I   John II   Alfred & Stephen (photo finish)

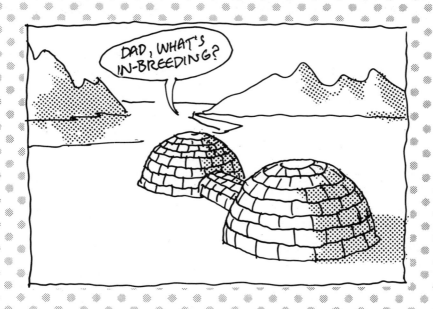

Sexual Snakes & Ladders

The aim is to get from the *Start* (Square 1) to *Bed* (Square 36) by throwing dice in turns. Bonus if someone you like gets there at the same time.

SQUARE 4
Go to disco Go forward 3 squares, then go back 3 squares, and repeat until it's your turn again.

SQUARE 6
Inherit £20,000 Advance 2 squares.

SQUARE 9
Develop cold sore Miss a turn while you learn convincing explanation of how cold sores differ from genital herpes.

SQUARE 14
Enter a nunnery Go back to Square 1 (if a woman); advance one square (if a man).

SQUARE 19
Get a reputation for sexual licence Go back one square (if a woman); advance one square (if a man).

SQUARE 22
Your breasts grow to the size of water melons If a woman, have an extra throw; if a man, go back to Square 1 and start again as a woman.

SQUARE 27
You become bi-sexual Your chances double; all subsequent throws count twice.

SQUARE 31
Your boyfriend/girlfriend/pet dog marries someone else Miss a turn while you work out whether they're just playing hard to get.

SQUARE 34
You lose all interest in sex Remain on this square until someone else lands on it to revive your appetite.

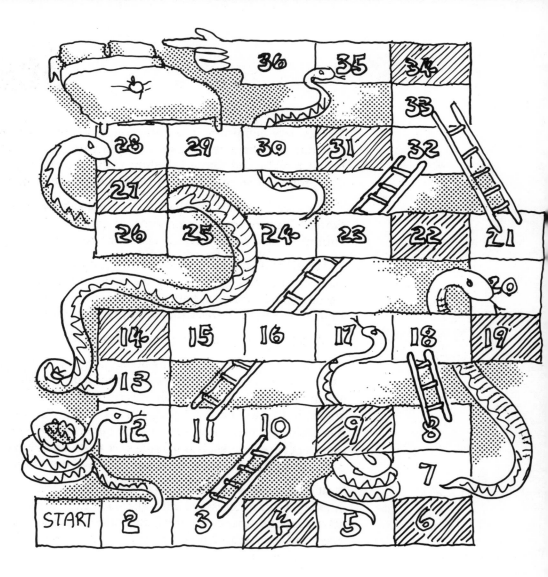

Sex:

Morals defy definition. They are 'concerned with goodness or badness of character or disposition, or with the distinction between right and wrong; dealing with regulation of conduct; founded on moral law' (*Concise Oxford Dictionary*).

They reached their zenith in the Victorian age, and like the British Empire and the practice of putting children up chimneys have been in relative decline ever since.

Morals regulate the readiness with which we have sex with people, and however free of them we may think we've become, they have a habit of re-emerging at awkward moments. In this respect they're rather like crabs.

Morality varies according to circumstances.

Julie from Solihull, for instance, may let Kevin from Wolverhampton go no further than the 'light petting' stage when they meet at a disco in Birmingham on a Saturday night; but when she's on holiday in Corfu she's happy to let Dimitriou go the whole way, having taken suitable precautions of course . . . such as making sure that Dimitriou's wife who cleans the villa they're staying in is well out of the way.

It's all to do with the sun . . . the sand . . . the carefree holiday atmosphere . . . and the fact that Dimitriou is dark-skinned, muscular and handsome, whereas Kevin is pale and spotty and wears a yellow anorak with 'Up the Wolves' on the back.

The Moral Dimension

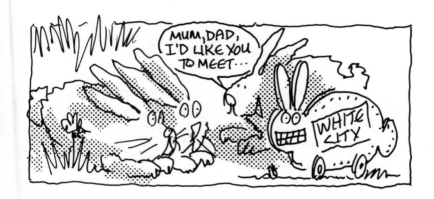

(Sun, sea and sand can in fact do a lot for your sex life . . . unless of course you have a lisp.)

Overleaf is a diagram showing the different moral codes impinging on the sex lives of two people.

(1) could be either a primitive stone age thug . . . or someone who hangs around the Hippodrome on a Friday night.

(2) might be the son or daughter of a Victorian parson living in a rural village near Tunbridge Wells.

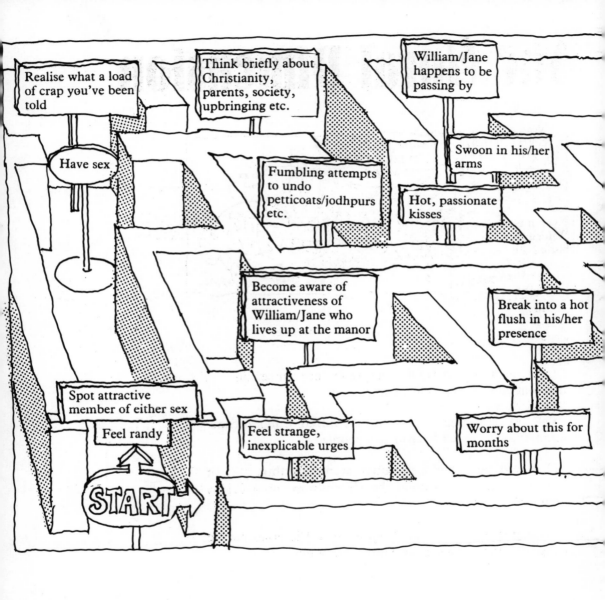

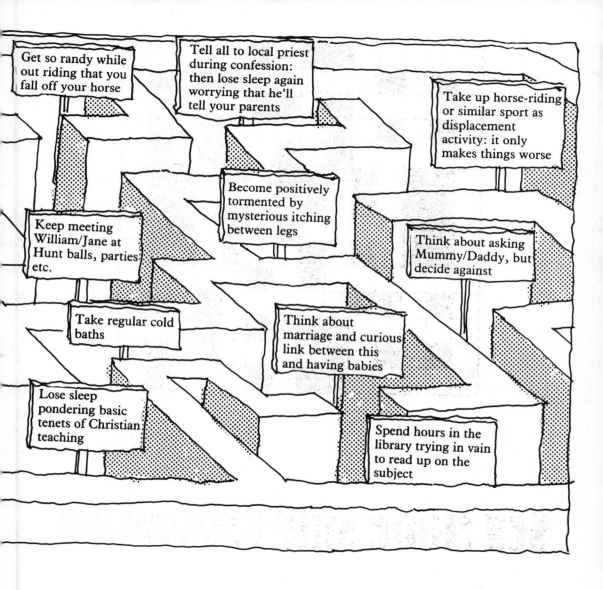

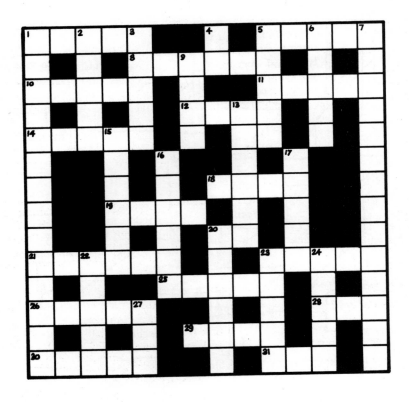

Sex Made Silly Crossword

Across

1/ Cuckold's dilemma. (5)
5/ Nonsense word used to fill blank spaces in ill-thought out crossword. (5)
8/ Noah returned what men and women both desire on both sides of the road. (4, 2)
10/ A Spanish cat in East Africa. (5)
11/ A nasty discharge, probably from an Italian. (5)
12/ Period before pregnancy. (4)
14/ King on top of mountain looks provincial. (5)
18/ Little Richard made this close to Great Balls of Fire. (4)
19/ Times 6.25, this makes a man average. (4)
20/ Tension sometimes follows this head of state. (2)
21/ They hang around in cowsheds. (6)
23/ Servant chops veals. (5)
25/ Labia majora majora. (5)
26/ These breasts are 21/. (5)
28/ This juice is a retrograde step in France. (3)
29/ Aphrodisiac after a gin. (4)
30/ Church is silent in the middle of status symbol. (5)
31/ Female half-brother. (3)

Down

1/ Really use the ox, bizarre, but not the way gays and lesbians do things. (14)
2/ Boy received and understood sexual act. (5)
3/ She has two litres and the perfect shape for an ear. (5)
4/ The inherited instinctive impulses you will find in a widow. (2)
5/ I get out of unisex and make less sexy. (5)
6/ A West Indian spiny cactus could be a penis substitute. (5)
7/ A place to pay to have sex with Ivy, and you can put your foot in it. (7, 7)
9/ Right, a Spanish cry is a part to play. (4)
13/ I mix with muted characters and so produce boredom. (6)
15/ A moral failing at the end of an advertisement is the result of expressing an opinion. (6)
16/ Mix up cars with Mississipi shortly and you end up with an attitude of mind that hates some people. (6)
17/ Head case. (5)
20/ Prigs first, softly rude second. (6)
22/ Gold in dick with the end cut off. That's some column! (5)
23/ Green cormorant has sex on more than one occasion? (5)
24/ Bottoms seen in bear's escape route. (5)
27/ Many go from meat but still put food in the mouth. (3)

*Solution on p. 96

porn porn porn porn porn porn porn porn porn porn

The word 'pornography' derives from two Greek words, (1) meaning whore or prostitute, (2) meaning to draw or depict; hence its modern English meaning, i.e. anything Paul Raymond can make money out of.

Pornographic magazines, films and videos are graded according to the hardness or softness of their core.

Warning: **The material below is of an 'adult' nature . . . i.e. designed for adolescents.**

Soft core porn Smiling near-naked girls are photographed with a soft focus lens in dull surroundings, such as on a beach, or on page 3 of a tabloid newspaper.

Very soft core porn Girls are shown singly or in pairs with little or no clothes on. Inanimate objects are positioned to conceal anything particularly naughty or interesting to the sensation-seeker. Some private parts are painted out with an air-brush.

Very very soft core porn Partly clothed girls are shown behind the hedge at a traction engine rally, holding a blown-up model of a speech by Mary Whitehouse.

Hard core porn Naked girls reclining on piles of half bricks and lumps of concrete.

Very hard core porn Generally unavailable in this country, since it tends to get seized at Tilbury docks by eager customs officials on its way over from Sweden or Denmark. Though why the customs officials can't queue up for it in their local newsagents like everyone else I fail to understand.

Porno Filth: Quest

(By kind permission of *Maypole* magazine.)

Quest   So just tell us about you and Paul in your own time . . . in your own words.
Interviewee   Thanks. Well, when I left college . . .

Q   Oh, just get on with the bit about you having it off with your neighbour while your husband was away on business in Coventry.
I   Hang on. *I'm* telling this story.

Q   Sorry.
I   Well, my husband was away on business.

Q   In Coventry.
I   Yes, all right!

Q   Sorry.
I   Well, that evening I was really looking forward to a quiet night in, relaxing in front of the television. I never thought it would turn out like it did!

Q   Shagging your next door neighbour?
I   Don't interrupt!

Q   Sorry.
I   Anyway, I had a shower, poured myself a drink and settled down to watch the telly, wearing only my flimsy dressing gown.

Q   Tell us about your ample breasts.

I   I've got two of them and they're on the front of my body.

Q   OK—get on with the story.
I   Well, I was watching this really interesting telly programme when all of a sudden a giant beanstalk shot up through the carpet right in front of the television.

Q   Were you surprised?
I   Very.

Q   What did you do?
I   Well, if I wanted to carry on watching TV I'd have to chop the beanstalk down. But I couldn't do it on my own. I'd need a man.

Q   So you got your neighbour round and gave him one.
I   This is *my* story!

Q   Sorry.
I   So I phoned next door. Paul answered the phone. 'Oh, hello Amelia. I suppose you want to talk to Susan . . . I'm afraid she's not here at the moment. She's gone away on business.'

Q   To Coventry.
I   Don't interrupt. So I told him of my predicament and asked him to come round. The last thing I said to him was, 'Don't forget to bring your big hard chopper.' I was embarrassed when I put the phone down and realised my *double entendre*. I'd meant his axe, of course.

Q   And what did he bring round?
I   His helicopter. Anyway, I was really embarrassed when

42

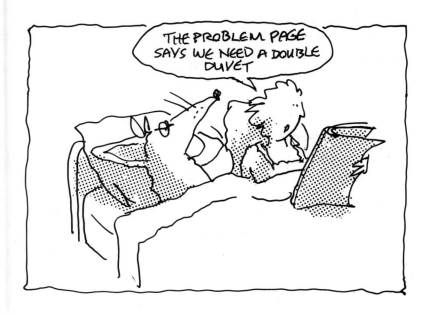

he came in. It all seemed so unlikely! My husband away
. . . Paul's wife away . . . and a giant beanstalk appearing
in my front room. It seemed so far-fetched. I'm sure he
thought I was trying to seduce him.

Q Tell me about his penis.
I You've got a one-track mind!

Q Sorry.
I Anyway, he started chopping down the beanstalk. I
thought it must be thirsty work so I offered him a drink. I
had some cold beers in the fridge. Anyway . . . it wasn't
my night, because as soon as I bent down to get the beers
out, my dressing gown fell open revealing everything.

Q   Have we got to the dirty bit yet?

I   Hang on, let me finish my story. Well, he obviously noticed because I saw the enormous bulge in the front of his trousers. He saw me looking. 'I suppose you're wondering about the enormous bulge in the front of my trousers,' he said, shyly. 'Well, it is rather big,' I replied. 'It's a bag of coal,' he said. 'Oh yes?' I said incredulously. 'Show me!' And he did!

Q   Was it a bag of coal?

I   Of course not. It was a bag of anthracite.

Q   What happened then?

I   We had sex lots of times and my husband came home from Coventry right in the middle of it.

Q   What did he do?

I   He was a management consultant.

Q   No, what did he do when he discovered you and Paul at it?

I   He screamed and said, 'Ah, I've just remembered where I put those magic beans.'

Q   Would you like to tell us about the juicy aching desire between your legs?

I   No, I've got to go to the post office.

Q   Thank you for talking to us.

I   My pleasure.

Two Martians landed on Earth and decided to try to find out something about the sexual mores of the English. As luck would have it they happened upon a liberated married couple on a housing estate in Carshalton who agreed to do a bit of wife-swapping.

The wife went to bed with the male Martian. She was looking forward to this extremely close encounter and was very disappointed when she saw what a small willy he had.

'Don't worry,' said the Martian. 'Just twiddle my ears.'

She did this and his willy grew by six inches; then she did it again and it grew by another six inches. The wife had a marvellous time and, at breakfast the next morning, had a contented look about her. She asked her husband what sort of night he'd had.

'Terrible,' he grumbled. 'I'm afraid Martian women aren't up to much in bed. You know what . . . all she did was spend three hours twiddling my ears!'

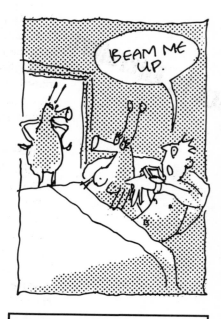

Did you know . . . ?
Some Spanish hotel builders can maintain an erection for as long as three weeks!

Sex in Literature

As all schoolchildren know, you get in trouble if you're caught reading porno filth in the classroom, but so long as it's an English lesson, and so long as the porno filth was written by a Great Poet or Novelist, you're in the clear.

Chaucer was the first really dirty author in the English language, and if he were alive today, he'd probably be struggling like hell to get out of his coffin. He used extremely naughty words like 'fart' and—even naughtier—'c--t' (sic) but because he could rightly point out that he had the first dozen entries in the *Oxford Book of English Verse* he was let off.

Besides, those were the lusty, merrie days of Olde Englande, when wine flowed a-plentie, wenches were considered rype for the pluckynge, and nobody had learned to spell.

Other English authors who didn't mind referring to the rude bits of the body by name were Donne and Byron, both of whom called a spade a spade, which proved very useful . . . especially when visiting the hardware store.

After that the Great Age of Prudery set in, and throughout the public libraries of England copies of the *Collected Works of Byron* were ripped open, and little stickers were stuck inside saying, 'This Poem Degrades Women'.

Nowadays it's all right to include the odd porno passage in an arty novel . . . but first you have to appear on tedious television book programmes, explaining that what you're actually doing is parodying, exposing and passing comment on the literature of sex, and if your readers happen to get a hard-on reading the stuff then it just goes to show what filthy minds they have.

Adolescence

In many ways adolescence—often described as a transitional phase between childhood and adultery—is the decisive phase in growing up, and it is during adolescence that we discover our sexual identity, and become aware of the sexuality of those around us.

This should be a source of wonder . . . excitement . . . that sort of thing. And yet for many girls and boys adolescence is a tormented and prolonged period of social awkwardness and sexual repression. For some, it's all over relatively quickly, and they are able to move on to a fulfilled and well-adjusted adult life. Others remain adolescent, psychologically at least, into their early and mid-twenties; they need sensitive, sympathetic support from family and friends. While some particularly pathetic characters never really grow out of it at all, and ought to be put in homes.

The adolescent charts show the various stages that a typical boy or girl can be expected to go through. But do remember that the ages specified are only averages and that it is perfectly normal for different phases of development to come either early or late.

If you think that charts of this sort are therefore perfectly useless, don't worry—that reaction is in itself completely normal.

Adolescence: Girl

Social Changes

Throw away childhood toys

Cancel subscription to *Jackie*

Tell Mummy to 'P★★★ off' for first time

Refuse to play 'Doctors and Nurses' with younger brother Andrew and tell him not to be dirty

Refuse to tidy up bedroom; put James Dean poster up on wall with bits of blue tack

Help yourself to contents of drinks cabinet

Develop crush on prefect in Sixth Form

Start wearing make-up

Go off Sixth Form prefect and decide you prefer boys instead

Physiological Changes

Early Adolescence

Slight bleeding

Period

Full stop

Discuss alternative forms of contraception with family doctor

Mid-Adolescence

First signs of pubic hair

Buy first bra

More pubic hair

Wonder what to do with bra

Late Adolescence

Adolescence: Boy

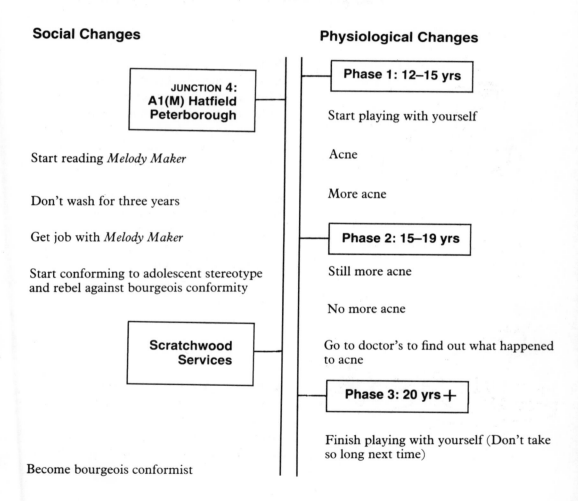

Social Changes

JUNCTION 4:
**A1(M) Hatfield
Peterborough**

Start reading *Melody Maker*

Don't wash for three years

Get job with *Melody Maker*

Start conforming to adolescent stereotype
and rebel against bourgeois conformity

**Scratchwood
Services**

Become bourgeois conformist

Physiological Changes

Phase 1: 12–15 yrs

Start playing with yourself

Acne

More acne

Phase 2: 15–19 yrs

Still more acne

No more acne

Go to doctor's to find out what happened
to acne

Phase 3: 20 yrs +

Finish playing with yourself (Don't take
so long next time)

Sexual Positions:

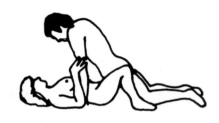

● **Missionary position**   So called because when Victorian missionaries went to Africa to spread misery and guilt, and to make the happy, civilised indigenous population filthy-minded and neurotic, they took the view that any other position was sinful.

The vicars willingly showed the natives exactly what to do, and, with the help of beautiful volunteers, they also demonstrated all the other positions which were banned . . . just in case the natives had forgotten.

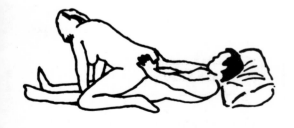

● **Reverse missionary**   Basically the same as the 'missionary', though having the woman on top, sitting astride the man, is thought to be a sign of female liberation and dominance. It also means she can keep an eye on the cooking.

A Handy Guide

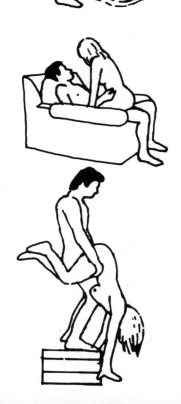

Doggy position   So called because it represents the favourite position of Archduke Doggy the Fourth, one of the ancient rulers of Zambonia. He liked to do it this way because it enabled him to rest a book on the girl's shoulders and read.

● **Armchair position**   Equal enjoyment for both partners as they can *both* read a book while doing it.

● **Impossible position**   Can only be done when one of the partners is abnormally short or tall, or when there's a cardboard box available. This makes for easy contraception—just as the man is about to come you kick the box away.

51

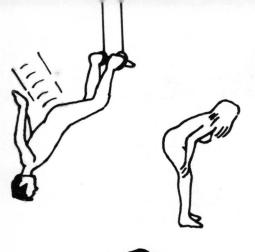

● **Just showing off position** Much easier to manage if the man is extremely strong and fit and the woman is tied to an airship.

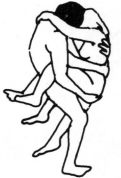

● **Is there somebody else position**

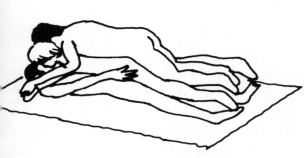

● **Submarine sandwich position** One for the keen, adventurous and athletic. We recommend that you have a doctor, a lawyer and a crane driver on stand-by before attempting it.

● **Wheelbarrow position** You can have it off as you go round the supermarket and load the shopping onto your wife's back.

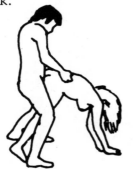

● **I wasn't expecting you back so early position**

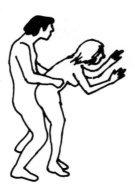

If the basic sexual positions still don't satisfy you and your partner, why not try some of these *Sex Made Silly* alternatives:

● **Thatcherite position** Woman gets on top and stays there for about ten years.

● **Soixante-neuf** Couple make love in any position they like while drinking a bottle of vintage red Burgundy; *or* dirty old man on top, little French girl underneath.

● **Dead hamster position** Couple astride each other on top of cushion, underneath which pet hamster has gone for a nap.

● **Hiatus position** Woman sits with legs apart on large cushion. Man squats in front and gradually edges between her thighs. Woman places leg over man's shoulders, gradually lowers her head then rotates her body through 180 degrees. Called 'hiatus' from the pause which now follows while they work out what to do next.

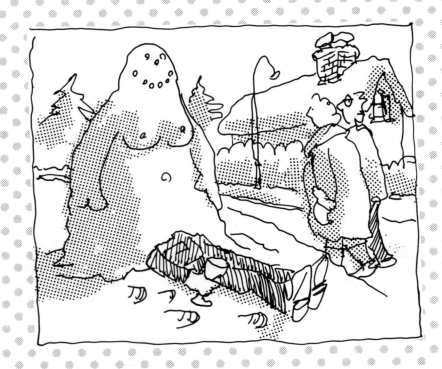

Foreplay

In many ways the act of sex is similar to having a meal. When we first get together with a new partner we go for a full-scale five-course blow out:

Hors d'oeuvre	**Heavy petting**
Soup	**Foreplay**
Main course	**Intercourse**
Dessert	**Post-coital cuddle**
Brandy	**Cigarette**
Ask for bill	**Ask for Bill**★

(★can cause problems if you're sleeping with Jim)

Then we begin to shorten the process, lopping off a course here and a variation there, and the build-up to sex gets quicker and quicker until we're left with:

Big Mac	**'Quickie'**
Chips	**Cigarette**

This is a shame, because foreplay is one of the most rewarding and important elements of sex. Without foreplay couples wouldn't be able to show their affection for each other in quite such a personal and individual way. Without foreplay it wouldn't be possible to introduce those important little variations into sex which keep the excitement up when the novelty has worn off. And without foreplay . . . let's be honest . . . the whole thing would only last about ninety seconds.

What to do . . .
Rub
Stroke
Tickle
Put your left leg in
Left leg out
Do the hokey cokey and
shake it all about

What to concentrate on . . .
Neck
Breast
Legs
Stuffing

What not to concentrate on . . .
Ankles
Elbows

That nasty damp patch
on the ceiling you've just
noticed

What to say . . .
'I love you'
'Mmmm . . . yummy'
'Oh . . . oh yes!'
'Lower . . . lower!'
'Harder . . . harder!'

What not to say . . .
'Are you in?'
'Stop calling me Elvis!'
'Will you take a cheque with a
banker's card?'
'Was that it?'
'Hurry up—I have to get off
at the next stop'

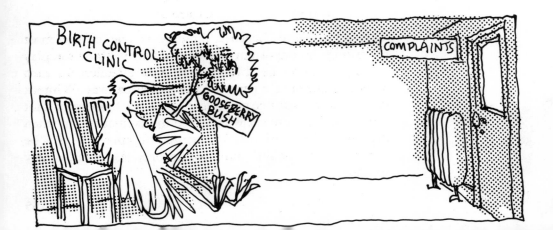

GETTING TO KNOW THE HUMAN BODY

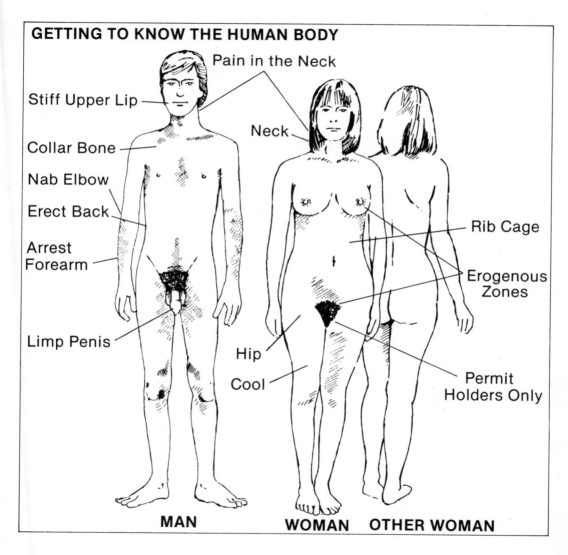

Pain in the Neck

Stiff Upper Lip

Neck

Collar Bone

Nab Elbow

Erect Back

Arrest Forearm

Rib Cage

Erogenous Zones

Limp Penis

Hip

Cool

Permit Holders Only

MAN **WOMAN** **OTHER WOMAN**

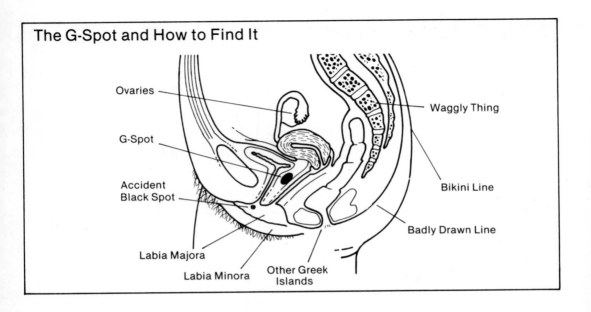

The G-Spot and How to Find It

- Ovaries
- G-Spot
- Accident Black Spot
- Labia Majora
- Labia Minora
- Other Greek Islands
- Waggly Thing
- Bikini Line
- Badly Drawn Line

If necessary, use this illustration as reference.

Premature Ejaculation

Not to be confused with *immature ejaculation*, i.e. reaching orgasm before the age of six.

Serious sufferers of premature ejaculation come to a climax within a few seconds of commencing sexual intercourse. Very serious sufferers will ejaculate even before getting into bed, and very very serious sufferers will come as they leave the house on the way to pick up the girl.

Most men grow out of this problem and then find they can keep going until the cows come home (or longer, unless they find cows particularly stimulating).

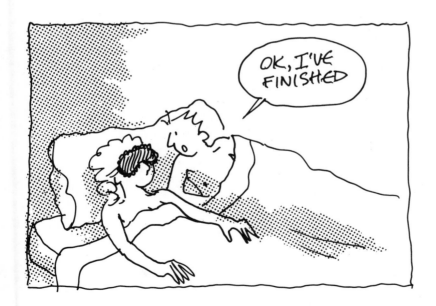

If it remains a problem you can try spraying your penis with specially made products such as Stud, Plonger, Airwick or Superglue. These will have one of two effects: (1) Stop you coming early (2) Make your testicles fall off. Both solve the problem effectively.

Another very good way to prevent premature ejaculation is to think of something mundane or particularly unerotic while in the early stages of intercourse. A doctor friend of mine used to think about what he had for breakfast and this helped him to restrain his excitement quite successfully. But he had an unfortunate experience in a hotel one morning when the waitress brought breakfast and he came all over his eggs and bacon.

Or, on the other hand, you could think of something dull while you're on the job and there are plenty of dull things on the planet: cricket, angling, brass bands, Sundays, answer-phone machines, books about sex, cricket, angling and brass bands. Mind you, thinking too hard about cricket might spoil your performance when halfway through the act you discover you're still wearing a box. Incidentally, if you do find cricket rather dull it can be cheered up by thinking about sex while you're playing it (see premature dismissal, leg-over-before-wicket etc.).

THE GRAPH OF THE ORGASM

PREMATURE ORGASM

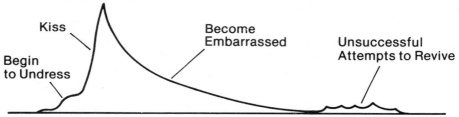

Begin to Undress

Kiss

Become Embarrassed

Unsuccessful Attempts to Revive

TYPICAL ORGASM

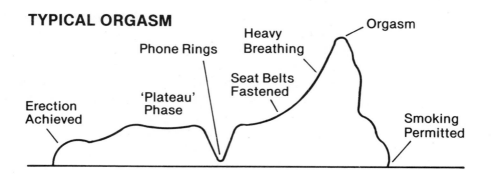

Erection Achieved

'Plateau' Phase

Phone Rings

Seat Belts Fastened

Heavy Breathing

Orgasm

Smoking Permitted

SWISS ALPS

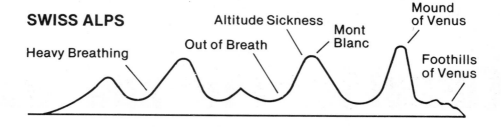

Heavy Breathing

Out of Breath

Altitude Sickness

Mont Blanc

Mound of Venus

Foothills of Venus

We all know how deeply satisfying sex can be when you do it with someone you love, someone you respect, someone you've committed the rest of your life to; though persuading the three of them to get into bed with you at the same time can be quite a problem.

There's no substitute for mutual understanding built up over many years' experience and for a deeply felt perception of your partner's individual needs, as my wife will confirm . . . and indeed, as any of my ex-wives would confirm as well.

But what of casual sex? In this permissive age we can find ourselves hopping into bed with someone we don't really know from Adam . . . as a matter of fact, it *is* Adam . . . well what's happened to Fiona, then? . . . that's a point . . . didn't I see her leaving the room with Hugo? . . . Hold on a minute . . .

Now where was I? Ah, yes. Casual sex. You know what it's like (at least Hugo and Fiona know what it's like). You think it's going to be the most earth-shattering experience, and then just as you get down to business you find that you've:

● come over all embarrassed
● come all over the bedspread
● can't seem to come at all.

Even if you safely negotiate the actual sex act, you've got what is arguably the most awkward phase: the *post-coital hiatus*.

Casual Sex: Pros and Cons

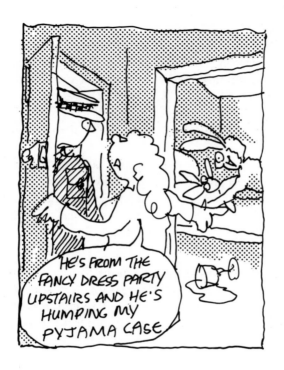

There are two basic rules for getting through this stage:

(1) Remain facing your lover. Resist the temptation to turn over and stare at the wall . . . however much the wall turns you on.

(2) Say something intelligent and original. This is surprisingly difficult since virtually all the different possibilities have been tried. Here are a few ideas:

● 'Mmm . . . Wow!'
(Indicative of the fact that you've been left speechless by the sheer wonderfulness of it; *or* of the fact that it was so mind-numbingly mediocre that you can't find words to describe it.)

● 'Hey! Let's still be friends' *or* 'That's the best exercise I've had in weeks.'
(Light-hearted, jocular remarks designed to bridge that gap between post-coital pregnant pause (*sic*) and return to everyday conversation; the danger is that you'll sound such a crass idiot saying these things that your partner will promptly get dressed and leave.)

● 'Don't worry—I'm not one of those crass idiots who can't resist spoiling what's really a very special moment . . . but that's the best exercise I've had in weeks.'
(Amounts to the same thing, though it's always possible your partner will have fallen asleep before you reach the end of the sentence.)

● 'Do you need a tissue?'
(Straightforward, practical and really quite tactful.)

● 'Were you safe? Bit late to ask, I suppose.'
(Straightforward and practical)

● 'If my mother could see me now, she'd have extremely good eyesight!'
(Straightforward.)

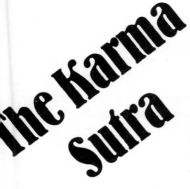
The Karma Sutra

The famous second-century manual of sexology by Vaatsyaayana entitled the *Karma Sutra* has long been considered the 'bible', if one may use that word, of liberated sexuality and erotica.

In fact, the *Karma Sutra* is an unintelligible, verbose heap of rambling drivel . . . about as sexually exciting as watching Ted Heath having a shit off the edge of his yacht. To prove this beyond any doubt we have included an extract from Vaatsyaayana's frightful book.

CONGRESS OF THE JADE MOON The man must wingle-wangle his lingam till the sun tinges with pink the sacred hill of bim bim. The lady must open her spicy papadam with the ivory bannister.

THE DRUMS OF JANGAPOOR For most perfect delectation of the love arts, the man, having eaten marbles with the one-eyed tiger, must dibble his boo boo with the leaves of the jelly biro. The lady, perfumed with a juice of thirty musks of brinjal, the 14 tears of smoked chimpanzee arse, and the 57 varieties of Heinz, must ballast her yoni with the ginger-flower of the buttock-tree . . . taking care not to ensnare her man's flopper in the holy mouse-trap of Biryani.

The lovers then dance to the drums of jangapoor splattered with the essence of moonlight, the spirit of cloud and the soiled kit of Raith Rovers 2nd XI.

YIN AND YAN The moon has a dark side. The moon has a light side. The light side is the murgh, the dark side is the Izal. Lovers unite in the temple of the Puckered Ane . . . where murg and Izal hold hands and swap tokens of love and lust and Marks & Spencer.

CONGRESS OF GIBBON MAN AND COMPOST HEAP WOMAN

Woman simmers the oil of fruitbat cheese till steam clouds dim the Sun of Great Ranjeev, the high priest of artificial hip-joints; she rubs the oil over Gibbon Man's bald snipers; he sings four hundred and five of the lust mantras of Blue Jay Way (leaving out 83 and 84 if pressed for time).

Here is one of the great pre-coital love mantras:

Hare hare hare
Hare rama
Hare rama
Hare rama
Hare hare hare
Hari shiva
Hari shiva
Hari shiva
Hari Kari
Hari Secombe
Hari Langdon
Hari Wilson
Hari Reynolds, Low mileage used cars, Ilford.

Hari buttock
Hari shinbone
Hari eyebrow
Hari minge.
Hari hari hari
Oi Oi Oi

Hari
Oi
Hari
Oi
Hari hari hari
Oi oi oi.

Who's your father
Who's your father
Who's your father
Referee
You haven't got one
You're a bastard
Who's your father
Referee.

Hari krishna
Hari krishna
Hari kirshna
Hari hari.
Om.

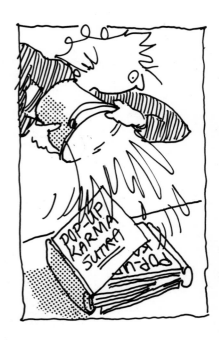

And here it is in its alternative, silent version:

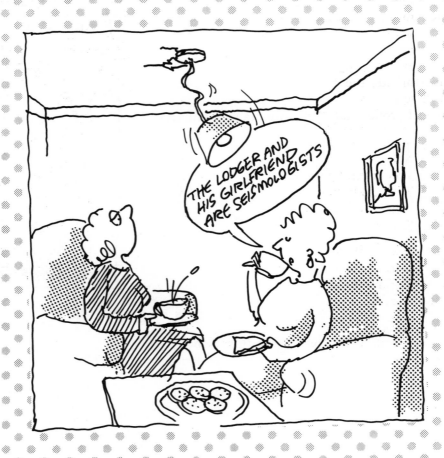

● ● ● ● ● ● ● ● ● ● ● ● ● ● ● ● ●

A little boy and a little girl are playing one day and the little boy takes out an apple and says, 'Look, I've got an apple.'

The little girl takes out two apples and says, 'Look, I've got two apples!'

Unperturbed, the boy takes out an orange and says, 'Look, I've got an orange.'

The girl proudly takes out two oranges and says, 'Look, I've got two oranges!'

A little hurt, the boy takes out his new pencil and says, 'Look, I've got a new pencil!'

'So what?' says the girl. 'I've got two new pencils!'

The boy is, perhaps justifiably, annoyed by this. Then he has a bright idea. He takes down his trousers and shows her his willie, saying victoriously, 'Look, I've got one of these!'

The little girl lifts up her skirt, shows the little boy her vagina and says, 'So what? I've got one of these. And with one of these, I can get as many of those as I want!'

● ● ● ● ● ● ● ● ● ● ● ● ● ● ● ● ●

Did you know . . . ?

According to scientists and doctors, men and women reach their sexual peaks at different ages. For men it comes early, at about 19. Whereas for women it's much slower to arrive, and of course some never reach it at all—they just fake it.

Agony Page

Sex Made Silly

Readers write in to the *Sex Made Silly* agony aunt Libby O'Leary, and her team of assistants reply.

Dear Libby,
> Can you catch VD from dirty lavatory seats?
> Yours, Dave (Hull)

Libby writes No, you can only catch VD from clean lavatory seats.

Dear Libby,
> Did Napoleon really say 'Not tonight, Josephine?'
> Yours Steve (Fareham)

Libby writes Yes, but unfortunately he was talking to someone called Madeleine at the time.

Dear Libby,
> Did cavemen really make love by knocking women over the head with a club?
> Yours, Reg (Huddersfield)

Libby writes Yes, hence the extinction of cavemen.

Dear Libby,

I know a lot of girls like a good ten inches, but I'm not folding mine in half for anybody.

Yours Lloydie (Vauxhall)

Libby writes *As the female porcupine said, 'It's not the size of pricks that matters—it's how many you've got'.*

Dear Libby,

I'm concerned about the size of my penis. My girlfriend laughs at it when I show her. It's just under half-an-inch long and half-an-inch wide. It's very embarrassing, and it's been swollen up like that for weeks.

Yours, Clive (Stoke Newington)

Libby writes *That's a ridiculously old and puerile joke. You should be ashamed of yourself.*

Dear Libby,

That's exactly what my girlfriend says when I drop my trousers.

Yours, Clive

Sex Made Silly Guide to

It's been said before that 'one man's taboo is another man's fantasy'. Also that 'one man's meat is another man's poison'. Also that 'one man's ceiling is another man's floor'.

Who is this man and why has he got such a muddled view of things? One thing's for sure, though. The dividing lines between what is and what isn't normal sexual practice have become more and more blurred in recent years.

We live in an era in which 'anything goes', and criminal prosecution for widespread bestiality and the practice of putting unmarried mothers in lunatic asylums are just a couple of the things that have gone.

Not that long ago, after all, it was thought that masturbation would lead to blindness. We now know that there is no truth in this at all—if there was, I'd hardGHKly be abRIHWle to typpppe thuissed ouut . . .

But enough old jokes, I hear you cry . . . or do I? I may be going deaf as well. We present below the *Sex Made Silly Guide to Exotic Sexual Practices*, as seen on TV (in *Play for Today*, late night continental films, *Blue Peter* etc.).

Bestiality

Bestiality comes in several forms:

(a) Sex between a man and an animal. This can lead to the man being sent to prison for life and the animal giving birth to a creature which is half-man-half-sheep (e.g. backbench Members of Parliament).

Sheep-shagging of this sort is relatively rare, and not to be compared with the good old days of the Wild West

Exotic Sexual Practices

when ladies were scarce and poking animals was the normal occupation (see *Harry the Horse, Buffalo Bill* etc.).

(b) Sex between a woman and an animal. This does occur, but only in the small, tight-knit communities of simple-minded folk who make pornographic movies . . .

(c) Sex between two different species of animals. This is forbidden by the basic laws of evolution, zoo keepers, David Attenborough etc. However, male donkeys (or asses) do crossbreed with female horses (mares) to produce mules . . . hence the unpopularity of donkeys with the owners of expensive female Derby winners.

If you think you have mild bestial urges, you should see a doctor or psychiatrist; failing that, try a sympathetic horse.

Paedophilia

'The vilest men in Britain—we name names!!' Many's the time we've seen this sort of headline. However, few people want to read lists of the editorial staff of one of the Sunday tabloids, so it's normal to turn the page and read about 'What the Rector got up to on the Boy Scouts' Summer Camp.'

Let's be quite clear about it: paedophilia is a messy and undesirable business. The psychological damage it can inflict is enormous. I mean, would *you* like to have a reporter camped outside your front door for months on end asking impertinent personal questions?

Sado-masochism

This usually starts in a harmless enough way with a little light spanking. There's no doubt that some people do derive pleasure from inflicting pain and having pain inflicted—within reasonable limits—and up to a point there's little harm in it.

But do for goodness' sake explain first to your partner what you have in mind . . . discuss it calmly and objectively . . . see what their feelings are and how far they're willing to go.

Then if they do object, you'll get all the more pleasure out of inflicting it on them anyway.

Anal intercourse

There's an old story of a girl who's about to get married, and her mother says to her, 'Whatever else you do, dear, don't ever let him do it the "other way".' 'What's the "other way"?' asks the girl, but her mother won't tell her and advises her to avoid it at all costs.

When she's married, she and her husband settle down to an enjoyable and highly fulfilling sex life. Everything is going marvellously and they both agree it would be hard to imagine a more satisfactory partnership.

The girl's curiosity has been aroused, though, by her mother's odd advice, and after a few months she begins to wonder exactly what the 'other way' is. One night after a tempestuous session of sex she's feeling so passionate that she plucks up the courage to suggest it to her husband.

'Darling!' she says. 'I hope you won't think me disgusting, but—just for once—shall we try it . . . the "other way"?'

'What!' he cries in a shocked tone. 'And have babies?!'

Most men start out in life by suckling their mother's nipples. This lasts for a few months and is altogether rather satisfactory; but then it comes to an end and there's a frustrating period of up to twenty years when it's impossible to persuade anyone to let you do this at all.

Oral sex

Psychologists believe that the urge to have oral sex stems from this breast-sucking phase. There are three types of oral sex:

(a) Fellatio

(b) Cunnilingus

(c) Talking about it.

(a) is mouth to penis (b) is mouth to vulva, and (c) is just mouth.

(a) and (b) are said to be very popular in America, where fitness fanatics have insisted on the introduction of low-calorie vaginal deodorants.

(c) is common amongst almost any all-male gathering, e.g. rugby clubs, TUC committees and Papal inquiries into birth control.

Homosexuality

Throughout history narrow-minded bigots have tried to impose their views about what is and what isn't normal on their fellow men and women. Sexual intolerance has been the cause of untold suffering and misery . . . any deviation from accepted attitudes has been met with suspicion and hostility . . . and those who practise it have become social outcasts.

Now at last a more relaxed climate is beginning to emerge, and it's finally becoming quite acceptable not to be a homosexual.

Stroll around the West End of London on a Friday

night, for instance, and you'll see men and women holding hands openly, even kissing one another in darkened doorways. There are even a number of 'straight' clubs where like-minded people can gather and mix socially . . . though they run the risk of being jeered at and even physically assaulted when leaving the premises late at night.

Prejudice against 'norms' runs deep; the very language we use demonstrates what a persecuted minority they are. To be homosexual, after all, is to be 'gay'; it therefore follows that to be hetero is to be depressed and miserable, usually about the fact that 90% of the attractive members of the opposite sex you meet at parties are so proud of the fact that they're gay.

Bigamy

The practice of having 2 wives at a time. In England this is a criminal offence punishable by having two mothers-in-law.

Polyandry

The practice of one woman having a number of different husbands. Much less common than *bigamy* and *polygamy*, it is in fact confined to certain Himalayan tribes and Elizabeth Taylor.

Incest

Often called the 'last taboo' though cannibals would dispute the claim.

Many regard incest as being second only to paedophilia as a repulsive sexual practice. In fact, on one occasion an entire village signed a petition demanding stronger measures from the Home Secretary. Signatories included:

- Tom Archey the gamekeeper
- Bob Archey the postman
- Archie Archey, Bob Archey's brother-in-law, and his wife Sam Archey
- Louise Archey and her four children, David, Richard, Emma and Mary
- the Archey family
- the village mayor (Josiah Archey)
- the village schoolmistress (Edwina Archey)
- secretary of the family planning clinic, Nora Featherstone (née Archey).

They were protesting about the only person in the village not called Archey, Jim Blackstone, who'd had his 'cousin' Lizzie to stay over Christmas.

Aids

Not to be confused with a type of biscuit you can eat to help you slim, this is a deadly disease which for some reason attacks groups of people connected by the letter H, e.g. Haitians, Haemophiliacs, Homosexuals, Heroin Addicts, Human Beings. Doubts are increasingly being expressed about the death of Harry Houdini.

In popular papers sufferers from this illness are always sympathetically dealt with under headlines such as NURSES WARNED AS GAY PLAGUE SLAYS ARCHBISHOP.

(*Text*: Nurses were warned not to read too much into claims by a tramp calling himself Archie Bishop that he was suffering from AIDS.)

A man was so depressed about being unemployed that he took a job at a zoo which wasn't doing too well due to its lack of interesting animals.

The job involved dressing up as a gorilla and spending all day in a cage behaving in a gorilla-like way. It wasn't well-paid but it was very easy and he quite enjoyed it.

His costume was that of a female gorilla, though, and one day the male gorilla started getting frisky. He tried to avoid the gorilla as best he could but the male gorilla was very persistent. The man was terrified and climbed out of the enclosure and along the walls of the other cages.

Eventually he lost his balance and fell into the lion's den. The lion glared at him. The man could stand it no longer. He ran to the cage bars and shouted, 'Help, help—let me out!' The lion leapt over to him and whispered ,'Keep your mouth shut or we'll all be out of a fucking job!'

Did you know . . . ?

The men of the Quezochitl tribe of Guatemala made themselves attractive to their womenfolk by smearing their bodies with crocodile dung. The tribe is now extinct.

Two nude statues, a man and a woman, which had stood in the park for over a hundred years, were scheduled to be moved to another park. The day before this was due to happen their fairy godmother appeared and said, 'You are soon to be separated, so as a special treat I'm going to make you human for one whole hour . . . and you can do whatever you like.'

The two statues wasted no time, and nipped straight into the bushes from where a lot of giggles and groans of pleasure could be heard. After half an hour they emerged looking pleased with themselves.

'That was fantastic,' said the male statue. 'Shall we do it again?' 'I'd love to,' said his friend. 'Only this time, you hold the pigeon, I'll shit on it.'

A little boy and a little girl were walking home from school after a sex education lesson which neither of them had fully understood.

'So what exactly is a penis, then?' asked the girl.

'I'll ask my Mummy tonight and tell you tomorrow,' replied the boy helpfully. But when he asked his mummy she referred him immediately to his daddy, who took his penis out and showed him.

On the way to school the next day the little boy, pleased with his newly acquired knowledge, told the girl. Taking his willie out, he said, 'A penis is like this only two inches shorter.'

SENIOR POLICE DETECTIVE SEEKS TALL DARK MAN (30s) WEARING BEIGE ANORAK AND BLUE JEANS. PHOTOFIT ESSENTIAL. BOX 421

OLD/YOUNG MAN/WOMAN SEEKS SKILLED, UNSCRUPULOUS SURGEON. BOX 933

MICHAEL TAROT. PROFESSIONAL CLAIRVOYANT AND MIND-READER. DON'T RING HIM, HE'LL RING YOU. BOX 167

OLD, UGLY, POOR, REJECTED, GAY GUY, EX-SCENE, LIVING GRAVESEND, SUFFERING FROM HERPES AND AWAITING AIDS BLOODTEST RESULTS SEEKS SOMEONE SLIGHTLY WORSE OFF TO FEEL SUPERIOR TO. BOX 825

21-YEAR-OLD GAY GUY, 6'2", MUSCULAR BUILD, SUN-TANNED, BLOND, HANDSOME, WELL-BUILT WHERE IT COUNTS, BROAD-MINDED, UNFUSSY, NON-SCENE, NON-SMOKING, NON-EXISTENT, SEEKS TO GET AS MANY PEOPLE AS POSSIBLE TO READ THIS AD. JUST TO TANTALISE THEM.

I AM A QUIET, LONELY 27-YEAR-OLD LIBRARIAN, NOT BEAUTIFUL, NOT UGLY, INTERESTED IN BOOKS, COUNTRYSIDE, KNITTING, TRAVEL AND EATING OUT. YOU ARE A BORED, CYNICAL SOD WHO'S JUST LOOKING THROUGH THESE ADS FOR SOMEONE TO LAUGH AT, SO PISS OFF AND LET SOMEONE LOOKING FOR A PARTNER HAVE A CHANCE. BOX 212

SHORT-SIGHTED DALEK SEEKS DUSTBIN FOR PASSIONATE SEX. BOX 576

SHY 33-YEAR-OLD DIVORCED ACCOUNTANT WITH UNUSUAL SKIN PROBLEM, INTO WALKING, READING NEWSPAPERS, RE-RUNS OF SGT BILKO, HALVES OF LAGER AND TALKING, SEEKS GIRL 16 TO 59 FOR MEANINGFUL RELATIONSHIP AND POSSIBLY MARRIAGE. IN REPLYING PLEASE STATE WHICH MAGAZINE, WHICH WEEK AND WHICH YEAR YOU SAW MY AD IN. BOX 123

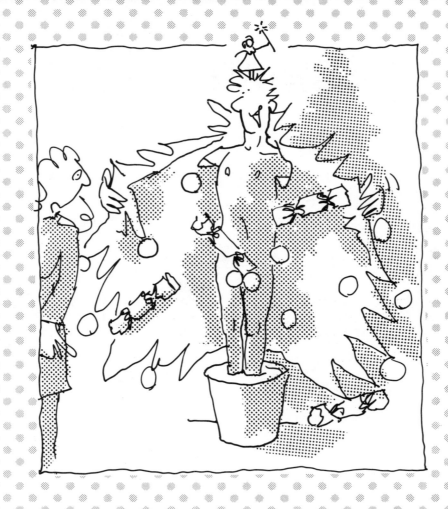

Contraception

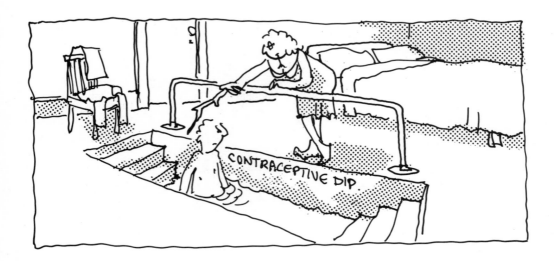

'The child is father to the man . . .'

W. Wordsworth
(whose ideas of birth control were rather sketchy)

People use contraception (literally 'contra-ception') when they want to enjoy all the pleasures of sex without the bother of having babies.

(By the same token they use artificial insemination when they want to enjoy all the pleasures of having babies without the bother of having sex.)

Although contraception has been around for centuries it's had a chequered and controversial history. The Roman Catholic priesthood, for example, remains stubbornly opposed to it, on the basis that since they aren't allowed sex at all, why should everyone else have the best of both worlds?

Attitudes to contraception vary in different parts of the world. In Ireland the Pill is only available to married couples. This is because the authorities mistook it for a fertility drug at a time when they were trying to boost the population to compensate for the constant emigration of Irishmen to become radio personalities with the BBC.

Whereas in other parts of the world, the reverse is the case and mass programmes for sterilisation have been initiated. In parts of China it's actually a criminal offence to give birth twice . . . particularly if you're a man.

In Great Britain those who want contraception can have it,

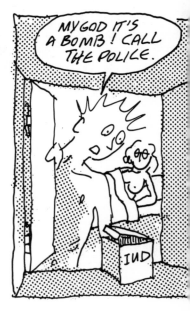

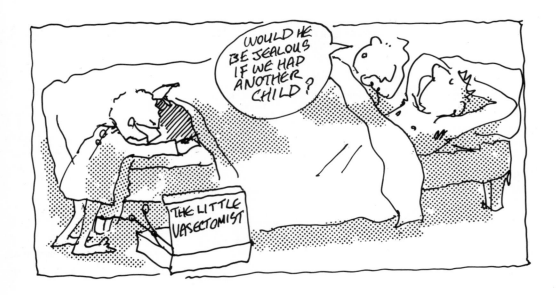

and some people believe that the same should be true for abortion, which should be 'available on demand'. Others feel that this really is going too far and that the woman should at least have to become pregnant first.

Most girls in this country first learn about contraception when they're twelve or thirteen, and all their schoolmates in the playground start talking about going to the doctor and being prescribed the Pill. This seems like a good idea, so they all follow suit and start taking it without their parents knowing.

As little as five years later they actually start having sex.

Contraception: the different methods

The Pill Usually made up of two synthetic hormones, oestrogen and progesterone. Best taken orally, as it can easily fall out of other places.

There is a story of a woman who goes to the doctor and asks for a 'contradictive' pill.

'God, you're ignorant!' he says.

'I know,' she replies. 'Two months!'

Rhythm Method A natural method in which by reference to temperature charts, phases of the moon and computer printouts, a woman calculates the times in the month when it is safe to have sexual intercourse (e.g. 10 days before ovulation, any time before puberty and any time after a vasectomy etc.). Advantages include approval by the Pope, easy to use for anyone with a degree in mathematics.

Side effects: pregnancy.

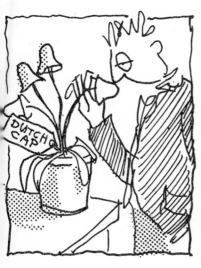

Dutch Cap Discovered by the boy who put his finger in the dyke. Ineffective if worn on the head (except as a way of putting men off).

The Sheath Main advantage is that it can protect you from certain nasty diseases (see under dirty lavatory seats).

Main disadvantage is that you have to buy it either from barbers' shops (otherwise known as contraceptive shops where you can have a haircut while you wait to be served), or from machines in public lavatories covered in such puerile

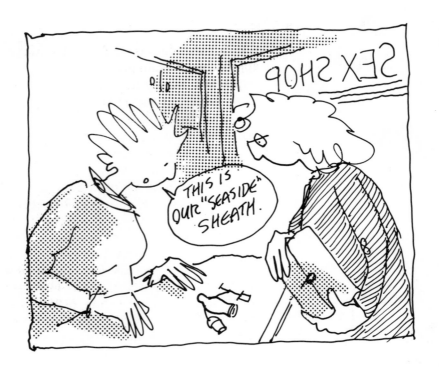

jokes as 'THIS CHEWING GUM TASTES AWFUL', 'SO WAS THE TITANIC', 'INSERT COIN AND TWIST KNOB' etc. etc.

The Coil   A spiral-shaped piece of metal implanted into the woman's body around the cervix by a doctor.

   Can be painful, but generally very safe. If a baby is born, it has a head in the shape of a corkscrew—very useful for opening the celebratory drinks.

I hadn't seen the cottage since I was thirteen, and now as I approached it again my heart fluttered behind my ribs like a caged bird beating its wings against the bars, knocking out the piece of cuttle fish onto that sheet of gritty stuff covered in old feathers and dried bits of budgie shit.

I wanted to sing with glee as I sprang from the taxi and ran towards the door. I'd come here to forget . . . and forget I would. Forget about Charles . . . forget about the anguish he'd caused me . . . forget the years of bitterness . . . forget the humiliation, the rejection. In short, forget everything.

'What about paying the bleedin' fare?' shouted the cab-driver.

'Oh, sorry. I forgot.'

The front of the cottage was enchanting—just like a picture postcard. I went round to the back of the house. On the walls in large letters was written 'Dear Ken and Vera, Having a lovely time. The weather is fantastic. Love Florrie and Arthur.'

Later that evening I'd made myself at home and was settling down in front of fire when the phone rang.

I was frightened at first because the cottage didn't have a phone. It did, however, have a tin-opener, so I answered that instead.

'Hello,' I said.

'Baaaaa baaaaa,' said a sheepish voice at the other end of the line.

'Hello?' I repeated.

'I'm sorry to bother you,' said the charming male voice. 'I'm your neighbour from Jasmine Cottage. I was just doing a spot of painting round the house when I realised I didn't have a stepladder.'

'Why don't you use a brush?' I asked.

'Do you mind if I come round and borrow yours?'

'All right.'

I was very nervous. I'd come to the cottage to . . . er . . . to . . . um . . . now what was it? Oh yes, I know—I'd come to forget. I certainly didn't need any male company. I was fed up with men.

No sooner had I put the tin-opener down than there was a knock at the door. It was him.

'That was quick,' I said.

'I came by poetic licence,' he replied. He stepped into the light.

'Watch out for the light!' I said. 'Damn! Too late.'

'Oh, I'm terrible sorry. I'll fix it—promise.'

I saw him clearly for the first time. I nearly fainted—he was the spitting image of Charles.

'I'm sorry about this,' I said nervously. 'Would you mind spitting?' He obliged. Amazing. Almost exactly the same as Charles . . . only his gob was less phlegmy and veered slightly towards the left when he spat.

We chatted idly for about half an hour. I really enjoyed his company . . . I hadn't failed to notice how handsome he was . . . Oh no, I was falling in love! How could this be? He was a stranger. I despised all men. I'd come to the cottage to be alone . . . to be free! This couldn't be happening.

'Do you want me to go?' he asked, sensing my discomfort. I wanted to say, 'No, stay . . . stay with me forever . . . hold me close . . . take me savagely . . . kiss me with reckless abandon.' I wanted to say all that but it came out wrong and I said, 'Oxford United are doing well this season, aren't they?'

He knew what I meant and took me in his arms. He kissed me. The touch of his lips made me feel heady. The touch of his head made me feel lippy. He was so much like Charles, I thought to myself. He seemed to be reading my thoughts . . . there was a slight pause . . . then he dropped his bombshell.

Half of the house was blown off and most of the outbuildings were irreparably damaged, but no one was hurt. We embraced passionately. Flames leapt through my heart and through one or two of the outbuildings. We were engulfed in timeless animal abandonment. We tugged at each other's clothes.

'Oh, Amelia,' he groaned. I sat bolt upright. I'd never told him I was called Amelia. I looked him squarely in the eyes. I knew something was wrong. He was so much like Charles. He knew I knew something was wrong.

'I knew there was something about you,' I said. 'I should have guessed—you phoning up the very evening I got here . . . making up an excuse to come over . . . looking so much like him . . . knowing I was called Amelia. So tell me . . . whoever you are . . . tell me the secret.'

He looked defeated. He lowered his head . . . and put it under the coffee table.

'You probably didn't know this . . . Charles probably told you he was an only child.'

'He did . . . you mean . . . ?'

'Yes . . . that's right. I'm Edna. His identical twin sister.'

X-Certificate

ADULT CINEMA COMPLEX Great Rogery Street.
£2.50 for three hours' non-stop entertainment . . . then
watch one of our films.

(1) EMANUELLE

(2) THE WIFE-SWOPPING PARTY

(3) THE VIRGIN SOLDIERS

(4) THE VIRGIN SOLDIERS' WIFE-SWOPPING
PARTY

(5) EMANUELLE TURNS UP AT THE VIRGIN
SOLDIERS' WIFE-SWAPPING PARTY

(6) THE VIRGIN SOLDIERS' WIVES TELL
EMANUELLE TO GET STUFFED

(7) SHE DOES

(8) SWEDISH SEX KITTENS AND NYMPHO
NIGHT NURSES DROP BY

(9) SO DO BLACK, YELLOW AND RED
EMANUELLE

(10) BLACK, YELLOW AND RED EMANUELLE,

EMANUELLE, SWEDISH SEX KITTENS AND NYMPHO NIGHT NURSES TAKE ON THE VIRGIN SOLDIERS . . . AND BEAT THEM 2–1 IN EXTRA TIME

(11) THE LOCAL CONSERVATIVE MP IS INVITED TO MAKE A SPEECH

(12) HE ONLY HAS TWO FREE DATES IN HIS DIARY . . .

(13) HALLOWEEN

(14) FRIDAY THE THIRTEENTH

(15) YELLOW EMANUELLE AND RED EMANUELLE TAKE A SAUNA TOGETHER . . . AND TURN ORANGE

(16) BLACK EMANUELLE TELLS EMANUELLE THAT SHE HAS SAGGY BOOBS, A FAT BUM AND DANDRUFF . . .

(17) THE BITCH

(18) A MANIACAL KNIFE-WAVING SEX KILLER IS ON THE LOOSE IN THE LEAFY LANES OF SURBITON . . . YES, IT'S THE LOCAL CONSERVATIVE MP TRYING TO FIND THE PARTY WHERE THE VARIOUS EMANUELLES, SWEDISH SEX KITTENS AND NYMPHO NIGHT NURSES ARE ALL MEETING THE VIRGIN SOLDIERS AND THEIR WIVES

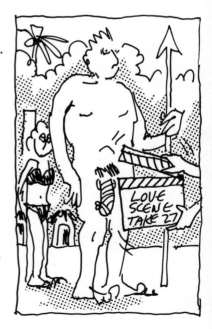

(19) HE FINDS THE PARTY AND DELIVERS HIS SPEECH (HALLOWEEN PARTS 1, 2, 3, 4, 5, 6, 7, 8 ETC.)

(20) MARY POPPINS POPS IN

(21) SHE IS SO SHOCKED THAT SHE REFERS THE MATTER TO MARY WHITEHOUSE, WHO CALLS THE POLICE

(22) THE POLICE TURN UP JUST IN TIME TO FIND THE VIRGIN SOLDIERS ABANDONING BLACK, YELLOW AND RED EMANUELLE, EMANUELLE, SWEDISH SEX KITTENS, NYMPHO NIGHT NURSES, THEIR WIVES AND MARY POPPINS ALL IN FAVOUR OF . . . MARY WHITEHOUSE

(23) THE LOCAL CONSERVATIVE MP TABLES A QUESTION IN THE HOUSE

(24) BUT THE ORGY'S GOING ON IN THE GARDEN

(25) RED EMANUELLE ACCIDENTALLY SETS OFF A CRUISE MISSILE STORED IN THE GARDEN SHED

(26) APOCALYPSE NOW

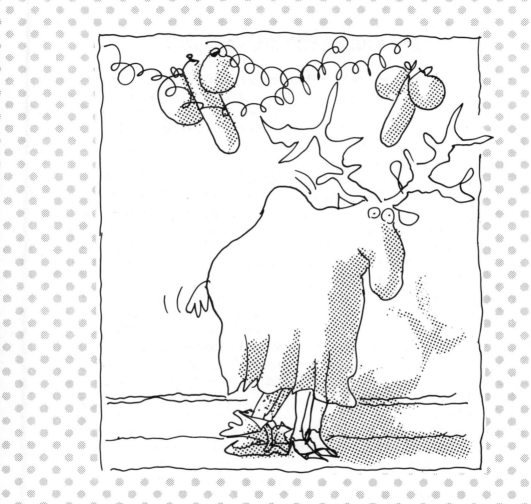

Glossary: The Sexual Act

More alternative expressions exist for the sexual act than for almost anything else in the language.

Take the simple phrase, 'He led me through to the bedroom, entwined me in his arms and enveloped me with his flaming passion.' This might otherwise be expressed as, 'We made love to each other', or 'At this stage sexual intercourse took place,' or—in legal parlance—'we shagged'.

Here is a list of the more common euphemisms (alternative ways of saying things) which are used to describe sex (physical intimacy).

Copulate Literally couple together, rather like railway carriages (hence all those films where they cut away from the dirty bit to a train steaming into a tunnel). The phrase 'Darling, let's go upstairs and copulate' is hardly one of the great romantic lines; on the other hand, it's probably better than . . .

Bonk Usually of other people, as in, 'Has Robert really been bonking Lucy? Good grief!' Since 'bonk' derives from 'bonkers', meaning crazy or mad, the implication is that Robert must be off his head to consider sleeping with Lucy, or indeed vice versa; which brings us to . . .

Sleep With One of the mildest alternatives available, and also one of the least accurate, since if Robert and Lucy have slept together it doesn't follow they've bonked, and if they've been bonking all night they can't have had much time to sleep.

Make Love 'Make love' is what you suggest to someone the first time you sleep with them (*sic*) and before you know them well enough to say, 'Come on darling—let's have a shag . . .'

Shag 'Shag' is a word for a type of sea bird, a form of tobacco and a make of carpet; hence its sexual meaning of having intercourse with a bird on a rug (followed by a smoke).

Screw Slang for 'prison warder' or 'worn-out horse' . . . well, it's obvious why the horse was worn out, though of course the prison warder denies everything . . . Anyway, in sexual terms, 'screw' is strictly speaking what you do to somebody who's using the coil (see *Appendix 2: Contraception*); not to be recommended to those who are prone to dizziness.

Roger   The chap who was bonking/shagging/screwing Lucy moments before Robert arrived, and had to make an undignified exit through the cowpats with his trousers round his ankles; hence the expression 'Roger and out'.

Fuck   An expression you use when you're typing out a manuscript and you accidentally press the wrong key on your electronic typewri

ter.

Know   People talk about knowing somebody in the 'Biblical sense', i.e. sitting up all night reading each passages from the Old Testament, or in the 'Shakespearian sense', same principle but marginally less boring. Not everybody's idea of a good time though an effective enough method of contraception.

❋ ❋

Outside Heaven there were two gates with signs over them: one said 'Queue here men who were dominated by their wives' and the other 'Queue here men who dominated their wives.'

At the first gate there was a tremendously long queue stretching for miles and miles; at the second just one ineffectual looking man. A friend of his in the other queue saw him.

'Hey, Gerry!' he called over. 'What are you doing in that queue?'

'I don't know,' he replied. 'Shirley just told me to stand here!'

Answers

Across: 1/Horns 5/Uxdmb 8/Hard on 10/Tigre 11/Salvo 12/Late 14/Rural 18/Dick 19/Inch 20/PM 21/Udders 23/Slave 25/Mouth 26/Large 28/Sap 29/Seng 30/Yacht 31/Sis

Down: 1/Heterosexually 2/Roger 3/Shell 4/Id 5/Unsex 6/Dildo 7/Brothel creeper 9/Role 13/Tedium 15/Advice 16/Racism 17/Skull 20/Prudes 22/Doric 23/Shags 24/Arses 27/Eat